AF334030

Tomorrow Is a Better Day

TOMORROW IS
A BETTER DAY

Dave Atwood

VANTAGE PRESS
New York / Washington / Atlanta
Los Angeles / Chicago

To my family and friends,
Dr. "T,"
and my co-workers at Monsanto,
without whose help I could not have made it

PREFACE

This book has been difficult for me to write. You see, I have multiple sclerosis, commonly referred to as MS.

It is basically a disease that affects the central nervous system, i.e., the brain and spinal cord. There is a destruction of myelin, a fatty insulation-type tissue that surrounds the nerves involved. The disease is characterized by a variety of neurological symptoms that could include one, a few or all of the following: difficulties with vision and hearing; dizziness; loss of balance; possible numbness in different parts of the body, as well as weakness and tingling feelings in different parts of the body; bladder and bowel dysfunctions; sexual dysfunctions; possible seizures and; rarely, dementia.

It can occur at any age, although it appears to hit females more than males, in the 20–40 age group. It should be noted that the severity of the disease varies in each case, and can run the gamut from benign to acute, the latter stage where patients go downhill rapidly and, in rare cases, may die within two years or less of related causes. The disease is wildly unpredictable and the future remains unknown.

Every person afflicted with MS will experience many of the same physical problems. However, the way each person will adjust to MS, and the way their families and friends will deal with the patient who suffers from the disease, varies greatly.

I am not the only one who had problems in learning how to cope with the illness. While I have the physical problems associated with it, I have to keep in mind at all times that my family, who I love very much, must adjust to those problems as well. It has been as difficult for them, at times, as it has been for me.

I sincerely hope that my observations, experiences, and thoughts that I convey throughout this book will not only help MS sufferers, but their friends, families, and loved ones as well.

"Hope springs eternal" is a saying we hear often and usually take for granted. It happens to be one of the mottos I live by. For we must always look toward God for help, as well as to our own inner strength in dealing with problems we face on a daily basis, with a disease for which there is no known cure. For only when we do this can we make sure that . . .

"Tomorrow Is a Better Day."

ACKNOWLEDGMENTS

There are many people without whose help this book could not have been written. I would like to thank the following people for their valuable contributions to this book: Henry E. Lattinville, M.D.; John Trotter, M.D.; Kongsak Tanphaichitr, M.D.; Gerard D. Ingenthron, director, Monsanto News Bureau; Yulinda K. Anders; Dave Watkins; Karen Lynn Trimble Dickey; Debra Ann Trimble Atwood; Kimberly Rae Trimble Atwood Martin; Donna Marie Atwood Piskulic; Diane Lynn Atwood Lifritz; Vickie Jo Atwood; Charles P. Hughes; Herbert J. Gebhart, Jr.; L. D. Monroe; C. (Cass) Kleyn; Naomi Williams; E. C. Makin; Dolores Le Grand; the National Multiple Sclerosis Society; Schnuck Markets, Incorporated; Dr. William Miller, American Red Cross, Missouri-Illinois Regional Blood Service; Sandy Ryan, director, Missouri-Illinois chapter Multiple Sclerosis Society; Mason and Gladys Stewart; Frank J. Atwood; and Shirley Atwood.

Tomorrow Is a Better Day

CHAPTER 1

"Multiple sclerosis."

The words hit me like the proverbial ton of bricks.

The doctor's words blurred as an entire lifetime flashed in front of me in three to five seconds. The seconds passed quickly as did the far-off words. Now I was focusing, and the words became more clear. Now I had some questions.

How serious? What stage am I in? Is it life-threatening? What about my family?

The focus was becoming sharper. Were the doctor's words really a surprise? Or were they confirming something that I had started to suspect some time ago.

Several instances came to my mind quickly.

There were occasions when I had lost my balance during the last several years. There was a fall downstairs. There was one heart attack, which came later. But my balance and heart strength always seemed to return. Then there were instances of blurred vision, and the headaches—oh, those painful headaches.

But now I was listening to a physician talk to me in layman's language—describing the results of a series of neurological examinations.

The construction of the medical history that was to follow me the rest of my life probably started in 1958.

1

CHAPTER 2

It was in 1958 that I first started to experience headaches. I was in the United States Air Force, stationed at Geiger Field in Spokane, Washington. I was nineteen years old.

The headaches were severe. They came suddenly, leaving bitter and constant pain lingering for about three days at a time. It was a particularly delicate spot to be in—I was performing Kitchen Patrol (KP) duty at the time, which obviously was not very popular, and a lot of the men in the same situation seemed to be suffering from a strange assortment of illnesses. It was easy to imagine that jobs such as scrubbing pots and pans, emptying garbage cans all day, and serving food to a whole base of men might make one search for an escape. I had the distinct feeling that the minute I went to see the doctor, everyone would assume that I was goofing off, perhaps trying to pull a fast one in order to avoid the unpleasant tasks; so, I put off the inevitable until the pain became intolerable.

The pain was such that in my worst moments I thought the only way to stop it was by putting a gun to my head and pulling the trigger. The restlessness I was experiencing would not allow me to sleep for any long periods of time. The headaches were like recurring nightmares. They lasted two and three days, leading to perhaps one day of peace, when I could feel like a normal human being somewhere along the line. And, just when I thought they were over, a sharp pain would hit me again. I could say they ran the gamut of degrees of pain, but how is it possible to differentiate between "terrible" and "*terrible*"? There really was no "in between" stage. Only when the headaches became more than I could bear did I decide to see a doctor, regardless of what my fellow workers might think.

My medical history was taken at the base hospital the following day, before tests were begun. Since I had no previous history of headaches or other medical problems, there did not appear to be anything out of the ordinary, or out of kilter—at least not on the surface. A spinal tap showed nothing wrong. The doctor gave me a dosage of ACR (known in the service as aspirin), and I was released.

It was only three short days later that a strange thing happened. I noticed that my left eye began to turn outward a few degrees. My vision was radically impaired. As I was performing duties of a search radar operator, I knew something was wrong immediately.

It was obvious to friends, as well as other people, as they noticed my expression was taking on a "wild-eyed" look. Objects near and far were hazy, and I experienced double vision sporadically. The base doctor had given me an eye patch, and I did indeed have a difficult time walking unless the eye was covered. (The purpose in using the eye patch was to strengthen the good eye. By covering the "bad" eye, the good eye was thus able to focus clearly.) The eye problem, combined with the searing headaches, finally convinced me that my condition needed further attention.

By the time I was referred to the base hospital for more tests, my eye had returned to its normal position. And, at this point, I was having no trouble with my sense of balance. However, no chances were taken with my health, and I was sent to an outstate hospital to receive the best medical treatment possible. (I remember thinking, rather pessimistically at the time, that the problem must have been extremely serious or else they would have kept me at the base hospital.)

I arrived at Letterman Army Hospital in San Francisco, California, in the summer of 1959, to undergo tests after suffering more symptoms. Doctors performed another spinal tap, in addition to a painful lumbar puncture (where dye was injected into a vein in the neck, allowing X rays to be shown of the head) and an arteriogram. It was first believed my problem was a brain tumor, due to the painful headaches combined with the more-recent turning outward of the left eye. I was scared and felt frightfully alone. My wife and daughters were in Spokane, and I prayed the results would not be as horrible as I imagined them to be.

The diagnosis was the same as it had been before. I left the hospital thinking how fortunate I was that the tests showed nothing; and, how extremely relieved I was to have found out there was no brain tumor. It still puzzled me as to what the problem was; but, I took the attitude, "If it isn't broken, don't fix it," and shrugged off the symptoms. When I returned to Spokane, the headaches lessened, and I regained control of my eyesight. I finally thought everything was going to be fine, because I was given no medication as well as a clean bill of health.

⌧⌧⌧⌧⌧⌧⌧⌧⌧⌧⌧⌧⌧⌧⌧⌧⌧⌧⌧⌧⌧

CHAPTER 3

I was stationed in the U.S. Air Force from 1956 to 1960. After my honorable discharge from the service, I headed back to my native St. Louis to search for a job. My wife, three stepchildren, and one-year-old daughter were to join me later. I was fortunate to land an interview with the Monsanto Company and pleased beyond words when I was hired the following week. I reported to work at the time as a production technician at the St. Peters, Missouri, plant. My job, which was to last there for three years, entailed all phases of silicon preparation. It took me two months to rent a house and transplant my family to St. Louis. Like all young men, I was glad to be out of the service and eager to begin my life as a civilian.

A new symptom emerged that put my optimism on the back burner, and I sought medical help again in 1961. I experienced a profound tiredness that I could not pinpoint or attribute to anything. I entered Faith Hospital in St. Louis, primarily to get some rest. Again, I underwent the usual tests, X rays, and blood tests. Testing was not extensive; and, again, the results were the same—nothing.

There was not another visible physical symptom until after my visit to the hospital. It came when my family and I went on a vacation to Casper, Wyoming, in the early 1960s. We visited a swinging bridge, suspended over a gorge, and naturally the family, in all their enthusiasm, wanted to try it. I followed reluctantly, and, lo and behold, yet another physical symptom hit me—I began to lose all sense of balance.

I also recalled another incident, coming out of the back door of my home in Wentzville, Missouri, heading toward the back fence. However, I never made it that far because I fell down. First I fell to one side, then to the other. I experienced a complete loss of equilibrium; and, to an outsider, I must have looked intoxicated. This, of course, put me into a state of shock, because it so closely followed the vacation incident. Unfortunately, it was a shade worse.

I could not walk, and it appeared that the multitude of symptoms I had experienced over the years was now leading to some kind of drastic conclusion—or at least I had the premonition that it was disastrous. The main problem was I had no idea what was wrong with me, the doctors had no idea what was wrong, and all of us were in the dark as to what should be done next.

I entered the hospital once again, and the same barrage of tests was performed. Both times I was given vitamin B-12 shots that perked me up and generally made me feel better. It was thought I had perhaps contracted a bad case of influenza; but, in my heart, I knew it was much more than that.

Other bodily changes were taking place. I began to drag my left foot, my left eye was drooping, and my speech was slurred (although I subconsciously wanted to attribute this to my rural twang). I should have anticipated the final results of all tests. A fortuneteller could not have predicted the results any better. All tests were normal in every respect.

⌧⌧⌧⌧⌧⌧⌧⌧⌧⌧⌧⌧⌧⌧⌧⌧⌧⌧⌧⌧⌧

CHAPTER 4

It was not until May 1968 that I was diagnosed as having multiple sclerosis, or MS. I suffered a repeat of the off-and-on symptoms, although not quite as pronounced this time. My family doctor referred me to Dr. Henry Lattinville, a neurologist (specialists who treat problems of the nervous system and its disorders). Dr. Lattinville made the diagnosis of MS. He based the diagnosis on the multitude of symptoms I was then experiencing and had experienced in the past.

After the initial diagnosis, a second opinion was received from another neurologist who confirmed that I did indeed have the disease. I returned to my family doctor with the news, asking him to take care of my medical needs. He assured me that he would.

From the point the diagnosis was made, my life took a 180-degree turn. I had never heard of multiple sclerosis before

6

and had had no idea where to go from there. My first reaction was shock, followed by disbelief. The next thought in my mind focused entirely on my family and what I needed to do to protect them.

I was assured that MS was not a communicable disease, and therefore no special precautions had to be taken. I wanted to downplay the disease, so no one would panic, yet didn't really know how my family would take the news or what their reactions would be. I wondered how in the world I was going to provide for my family, because the disease is one that becomes progressively worse. From where I stood, I seemed a doomed man. I also wondered how much longer I would be able to hold a job.

After I was diagnosed as having MS, I got in touch with the St. Louis Veterans' Administration. We agreed that I had probably contracted the disease while in the service, with the excruciating headaches being the first clue. I looked back on that time and wondered how many other people on that site, perhaps at a later date, might have contracted the disease.

And, I know that for whatever happened to me and my family after that, one thing was for certain—none of us would ever be the same.

CHAPTER 5

I had gone to work for the Monsanto Company in 1961, first as a production technician. Monsanto has often been referred to as a "people-oriented" company, and I can personally attest to that. I was comfortable there, even when it became apparent that my disease was becoming progressively worse. I was transferred to the Creve Coeur branch in 1964 and recall my first boss, Mr. Earl C. Makin, telling me, "David, you come first, then your family, then the Monsanto Company."

That phrase—stored in memory bank to this day—and my belief in the company, was proven to me immediately after it was ascertained that I had MS. I informed Earl of my situation after the disease had been officially diagnosed by Dr. Lattinville on May 3, 1968. It was his responsibility, in turn, to pass the information on to the personnel department, which he did.

The company did not put me out to pasture, nor was I ever made to feel out of place. I enjoyed my work to the fullest, and it was the one thing, with the exception of my family, that gave me a definite reason to get up every morning. Since the company also stressed pride, knowing that I had responsibility gave me the confidence I needed. I feel that sense of well-being is one of the reasons I am still active today.

Please keep in mind: Just because I happen to have MS, I am still a man in every sense of the word. I had had a family to support, and it was crucial that I was treated like every other man in the work force. I believe it would be difficult for any male to think he was in a position where he could no longer support his own family; perhaps I may be a little chauvinistic in that area, thinking of the man as the sole provider. But, I do know that when you strip a man of the dignity of doing his job to the best of his ability, something inside of him dies a little.

Earl was always understanding, and, believe me, on some days that was an understatement. There were periods when my eyesight was so bad that he arranged to have me do a different type of job, one where eyesight was not as crucial to actual performance or did not interfere with the necessity of the preciseness of the task. Earl told me to continue to work, as he saw no reason why I should stop. There were minor restrictions placed on me several years down the road, but until that point, I capably performed my job as a chemical research technician. Safety was the factor stressed the most in my position, as it was also stressed to other employees.

Management respected my judgment in that I would perform to the best of my ability and not attempt jobs that I did not feel I could handle. I was also fortunate in that everyone kept a watchful eye over me.

My wife Shirley and I never fail to be touched when recalling a specific overture made by Earl and Mr. Rod Beckham, another one of my supervisors.

At the time I informed the company I had MS, both gentlemen took Shirley to lunch and assured her that my job was secure and I would not be fired. It gave her an enormous sense of relief to know that we were not going to have to worry about finances—a natural thought when you have six children to raise!

They assured her that they would do everything they could to help. I found out about this act of kindness at a later date and will always be grateful for the gesture—one that was above and beyond the call of duty of management.

⌘⌘⌘⌘⌘⌘⌘⌘⌘⌘⌘⌘⌘⌘⌘⌘⌘⌘⌘⌘⌘⌘

CHAPTER 6

I have always tried to work around my disabilities and was fortunate in that my boss was the kind of person who understood this and gave me many opportunities to prove myself. For example, I could build and operate different types of research apparatus and perform many types of analyses. In addition, I was allowed to set up and operate distillation equipment. For that reason, I have always tried to give more than what was expected of me. (Of course, I will admit that I still don't know for a fact whether this was because Monsanto was so good to me or whether I was trying selfishly to prove something. I think it was a combination of both.)

To an outsider, the office where I worked was actually a laboratory that had a "mad scientist" atmosphere—one straight out of a Frankenstein movie. There were tubes and wires everywhere, each of them leading to different places. There were many smaller labs contained within the major one, each used for different projects. Each of the projects, in turn, were carried out for different purposes.

At one point, my task was to put small stainless steel tubing into a system that I was building. The finished unit was to be put into a small laboratory. I just couldn't seem to make the connections, which had to be made by screwing metal fittings on to various connectors, because of the lack of hand coordination and bad eyesight I was experiencing at the time.

L. D. Monroe, the senior research technician, typified the many supportive people with whom I have worked with over the years. In cases when I got to the point where I needed "two good hands and two good eyes," L.D. was usually around to give me help and boost my morale. An understanding boss is vital, and support of co-workers is next in line to importance. The deadly sin of "pride" being what it is, I would often have difficulty asking for help, but these special people always magically appeared to help.

I informed my co-workers that I had MS after my boss had been told. The working arrangement resembled a small family atmosphere. They were concerned for my health, but in no way ostracized me or made me feel out of place. My family and I socialized with them before and after the MS was diagnosed. The friendships are as we have kept them today. It sometimes seemed ironic—on one hand, everyone pitched in to help when they were needed; but, on the other hand, they chose to totally ignore any handicaps I might have had.

The support of my co-workers meant everything to me, and they never missed an opportunity to show it. I tried never to take advantage of their kindnesses, but those special privileges and favors that made life easier for me will never be forgotten.

For example, it was not unusual to have a co-worker get behind the wheel of my car and do the driving duties when it was my turn to chauffeur the car pool. Even the personnel department cooperated by issuing a pass for me to park in the visitors' section of the parking lot when I was having a rough day. (There were no spaces for handicapped parking back then.)

There were many times while working that my life became loaded with frustration. Sometimes I thought of just giving up, as it would have been so easy. One can never tell what the next day will hold in the way of physical ailments for the MS sufferer. Instead, I would get a grip on myself and have a cup of coffee, or perhaps take a short walk. It was odd how the simplest of remedies would cure those negative feelings when they arose. Kind words from co-workers were excellent medicine as well.

There were other times when it would not be quite so easy to shake off momentary feelings of depression. These periods were usually short, lasting minutes or, at worst, all day. The most difficult times occurred when I would have to do something which required good eyesight or hand coordination, one or the other or both of which I might not have had at the time.

Frustration welled to the point where it became easy to

feel sorry for myself, and sometimes this depression was most severe. I coped with the longer-lasting depression by taking half-day vacations, choosing to stay at home. I would sit in the backyard, my mind blank. Sometimes I would look out over the yard, as if it were a freshly plowed field, with the good earth reminding me of soft velvet, a vision I had conjured from my childhood. These were times when I wanted to be by myself, and I expressed my depression to no one—not even my wife.

Occasionally, I would casually mention how I felt to a co-worker, but never elaborated. During those days, I also had a low tolerance for patience and became overly impatient with my daughters over insignificant things, which would ordinarily never bother me. However, as stressful as these periods were, I never once contemplated suicide.

The depression that I was experiencing was usually the end result of trying to perform a simple task and, in the end, not being able to do so. For example, at work I might be assigned the precise job of weighing chemicals into small amounts, some as tiny as 0.1235 grams, then putting these amounts into bottles with very small openings. This type of work would later be used in a research project.

There were times when I performed a job known as liquid phase work. A phase point was reached when enough liquid chemical was added to another, going one drop at a time.

It was vitally important to watch the solution carefully, as the phase point was obtained when the solution became cloudy.

I had problems with my vision and, at times, could not tell when this change occurred. It was necessary for me to ask for Earl's opinion, to make sure my work was satisfactory. It was not embarrassing to ask for help, but, I admit, wondering if my work was accurate put me under a mental strain. I often wondered if my bosses felt uneasy or questioned my ability.

If I happened to be weighing out liquids, I might be using a small pipette, a round glass tube graduated on the end, used for transferring amounts of liquids from one place to another. Since I only might be adding one drop at a time, in order to reach the proper weight, I had to be very cautious. Needless to say, this was quite difficult for me to do at times, since one had to possess good hand coordination and eyesight; hence, frustration.

Other times I might be running small stainless tubing to different parts of research equipment I would be building. I would put this tubing into a small area, one which might be hard to reach. At times like this, I would ask L.D. to give me a hand, but I would always try to accomplish the task myself first.

⌧⌧⌧⌧⌧⌧⌧⌧⌧⌧⌧⌧⌧⌧⌧⌧⌧⌧⌧⌧⌧⌧⌧

CHAPTER 7

At the time, it finally became quite clear to me that I had reached the point where I should consider retirement from Monsanto, for medical reasons—around the age of 42.

A definite incident triggered the decision. I had been in the middle of weighing different liquids into a bottle, then analyzing the liquid in the bottle. By knowing the weights of the different liquids, I would know what the percentage of the liquid should be. However, in performing this job, I came out with the proper weights, but inevitably it would turn out wrong. I found that as I placed one drop of liquid into the bottle, that bit of liquid would end up dripping outside the bottle instead of inside.

Mr. Bob Schultz, my immediate supervisor at the time, pointed out what I was doing wrong. I was never upset over constructive criticism about my work, but I do admit that I took the criticism personally, although it was never meant to be. I sometimes looked at it as a failure on my part. And ever since I found out I had MS, I have always tried to compensate for things I could not do well. It always seemed to be a personal failure on my part. There were times when I wanted to yell, "Hey, this is my body's fault—not mine! I'm not doing these things on purpose!"

I was forced to accept the fact that I could no longer perform an adequate job—something that I still have a difficult time dealing with. Besides my job, my dignity was at stake.

There were times when I reflect that perhaps my working years would have been easier had I asked co-workers for help more often. But, when you have a disease like MS, it makes you all that more determined to do things by yourself, with as little help as possible. Of course, I cannot overlook the fact that I am also a stubborn person by nature, and this combination sometimes leads to a dead end.

Retirement was something I knew would happen sooner or later, and, since I had reached that point, it suddenly became quite frightening. Bob Schultz offered me other possible job alternatives within the company, but I felt the strong need to retire. I had reached the end of my rope both physically and mentally.

⌧⌧⌧⌧⌧⌧⌧⌧⌧⌧⌧⌧⌧⌧⌧⌧⌧⌧⌧⌧⌧⌧

CHAPTER 8

I handled my upcoming retirement situation quite poorly at home. I made the terrible mistake (one which still haunts me today) of not discussing my intention to retire with my wife. Instead, I chose to tell her after I had already offered my resignation.

This was selfish on my part, but, at the time, I thought I had her best interest in mind.

I announced my retirement on Friday afternoon, and that same weekend we drove to the Ozarks (in Missouri) for a short vacation. It was not until we were driving home that I told her I had retired.

Shirley, needless to say, was absolutely furious and later told me that she would have slapped me had it not been for the fact that she was driving.

"It bothered me that I wasn't regarded as an equal in your decision," she reflected later. "You had already made up your mind, officially retired, and said absolutely nothing about it. I just felt that this was something which was a major decision and I was excluded from it. It stung me to know that you didn't trust me enough to let me participate in the decision making, or to talk things through with me first. In fact, I didn't even know you were thinking about retiring!"

You know, being a typical male animal, I just wanted to protect Shirley. I wanted to have everything under control—financially and otherwise. I can see that I was wrong and should have shared this with her; but, at the time, again, I let pride stand in the way of what would have been a rational thing to do. She really understood the reason I retired, but my judgment was poor in handling the situation.

CHAPTER 9

Unfortunately, there also came that point in time when I, myself, knew the MS was getting worse. I was drained all the time, both mentally and physically, and felt like I just couldn't carry on anymore. My vision was faltering, my balance terrible. I experienced a painful swelling of my heels and lacked hand coordination. And, no matter how hard I tried to make my work satisfactory, it just wasn't that way.

To give an example of the day-to-day confusion my illness created, I can remember writing a short note to a friend—one that was almost readable. However, that was only on one particular day. The following day, or the day after that, I might try and write another letter, and my handwriting might be atrocious, resembling chicken scratching. The problems with my hands hit all at once, catching me completely off balance. At breakfast one morning, I became frustrated when I could not perform the simple task of putting butter on a biscuit. I suddenly got the urge to rear back and throw it on the floor. Fortunately, I contained myself and nothing happened.

There were many day-to-day frustrations with MS. The simplest of the tasks become the most complicated feats. And, while my handwriting might have been bad on a particular day, I was fortunate in that I could walk a straight line.

It felt good to be able to walk well, even if it was only for isolated days, because, with MS, one never knows when a particular symptom will worsen.

I was referred to Dr. John Trotter, a neurologist at Barnes Hospital. I was given a neurological examination. He found me to be in stable condition and advised me to continue taking Prednisone pills. I had been taking the medicine to control eosinophlic vasculitis, and it helped the MS by controlling swelling of joints. I was taking an average dosage of 10 milligrams per day for a one-year period, given to me initially for recurring skin lesions. I also continued taking vitamin pills.

There are a few medications that help control the symptoms of MS, but there is no known cure for the disease itself. My days were like roller coasters—up and down, from one day to the next, with no advance warning.

Then something else happened. As I was leaving the doctor's office, instead of going to the front door, I thought I would take a short cut out the side door. When coming out the door, there was a stoop about four feet above the sidewalk, with stairs leading down to the walk. After getting out of the door, I suddenly realized I was in a bad situation. I could not get back inside the door, nor down the stairs. I was terrified that I would fall down the steps, and this was the type of feeling that completely paralyzed me. After being immobilized with fear for a few minutes, I finally got down on my hands and knees and crawled to the stairs. With much difficulty, I made it down the stairs to the walk. You can imagine how relieved I was to be able to get out of that predicament. This was one incident in my life that I will never forget. I still get goose bumps when I think about it.

I also became concerned about my overwhelming fear of high places—a condition called "aerophobia"—so much so that I finally went to see a sociologist at Medical Care Group of St. Louis—a division of Washington University—about this problem. I was concerned about it being mental in nature, but she assured me it was quite real. (Thank goodness I was not going crazy, although that too crosses my mind, even now!)

I reached the point where, when coming off a ramp from a highway, I became squeamish and remain so today—such is my fear of high places. I cannot park in a parking garage anymore. My left eye is turned outward just enough to make depth perception faulty. My eyesight is not strong enough, or I should say not finely tuned enough, to park in extremely close quarters. When driving an automobile, there is no room allowed for poor judgment with regard to eyesight.

No, I'm not able to drive much these days, and particularly not after dark. I have a moral obligation not to do anything that would place myself or others in jeopardy.

Hard-headed. Stubborn. Determined. Those adjectives fit me to a tee. I have never been able to get it through my hard head that I simply cannot do all the things that everyone else takes for granted—those everyday tasks, like carrying a cup of coffee across the room without spilling it, climbing a ladder to change a lightbulb, or buttoning a shirt.

Shirley often used to say, "David, you won't admit to yourself that you have MS."

She was right—in a way. There is no doubt in my mind that I have MS. However, what I have a hard time dealing with is the fact that no matter how bad the symptoms become, I keep thinking I can overcome them. Each day I am physically reminded that I have it; but each day I think somehow I can outsmart it. And, have never given up hope of scientists finding a cure, no matter how far into the distant future that day might be.

⌘⌘⌘⌘⌘⌘⌘⌘⌘⌘⌘⌘⌘⌘⌘⌘⌘⌘⌘

CHAPTER 10

I had no choice but to retire. During the period I was thinking about taking Medical Retirement from Monsanto, I also thought pretty hard about what I would do with myself after I actually stopped working.

This is a universal concern to all those who retire, as then, a person suddenly has an enormous amount of time available; but, it was particularly a great concern to me, because I never had the choice of activities open to many others. I had to think in terms of getting involved in things I was physically capable of doing, not necessarily things I would have otherwise preferred. For example, mountain climbing was out of the question!

No one wants to quit working and sit in a rocking chair thinking longingly of days gone by, and no one wants to turn into the stereotypical retiree who goes fishing every day. I have always appreciated the expression "If you don't use it—you'll lose it!"—this is especially true of retirement. And, since I was retiring at a relatively young age, it meant that I would have an unlimited amount of time on my hands.

So, what I wanted to do seemed quite natural—I very much wanted to do volunteer work and help other people afflicted with MS. But, first, I had to find the channels that would lead to this specific area. My work with MS patients was to come much later.

Before I retired, I also thought of hospital work; and, this was ultimately the course I pursued. Hospitals are always looking for good volunteers and particularly ones who have been through unfortunate circumstances themselves and can relate to patients who might have given up hope. I felt, by virtue of seeing me on my feet, being operational, it would be enough to let anyone who had the disease know that one can still function as a human being.

No one has to give up on life and quit doing things they enjoy. On the contrary, one is so much better off, both physically and mentally, to not give in to a negative attitude.

⊠⊠⊠⊠⊠⊠⊠⊠⊠⊠⊠⊠⊠⊠⊠⊠⊠⊠⊠

CHAPTER 11

The first place I performed volunteer work was Christian Northeast Hospital in St. Louis. My job consisted merely of talking to people and running errands for nurses. Later on, I started volunteer work at Christian Northwest Hospital in St. Louis, choosing the psychiatric ward, mainly because I felt comfortable with the patients, and there were more people I thought I could be of a help to, if even on a small scale. I decided to cut back to only one hospital when the stress began taking a toll on me physically. Specifically, the hospital consisted of four floors, and it became difficult to navigate myself from one floor to the next.

Unfortunately, the mental strain also took its toll and became too much to handle. For many people, it is easy to become emotionally involved with the problems of patients, and it is something over which you have no control. I found myself slipping into this category.

I continued my work at the American Red Cross Organization in Ferguson, Missouri, where I worked with the blood donors service department. This volunteer job gave me much satisfaction for three years. Basically, my job consisted of telephone work, calling people who had previously given blood, and asking them to repeat. Hospitals are always in need of donors, and this was a responsible position for me to hold.

Today, my volunteer work consists of giving two hours of service each week at the MS Society in St. Louis; two hours each week at Christian Northwest Hospital; and, up until December 1984, three hours each week at the American Red Cross.

I like to tell people of my philosophy, which is to never give up—always keep presenting reasons and devising goals and challenges to keep your life meaningful. I have to remember this at all times, because there are so many dark days when I'm hit with a multitude of physical problems. My balance might be bad one day, and the next day my arm might be numb. The following week perhaps my entire leg might be numb; and, sometimes without warning, my body begins to jerk uncontrollably, causing me to lose control of my muscle coordination. In the face of these grim realities, which I cannot control, I must remind myself of that philosophy of mine over and over.

We all need a purpose to our lives, and volunteer work has given me that unique meaning, a purpose to get up in the morning, knowing I have something meaningful to do and somewhere to go. My children are now grown and my wife is self-sufficient. I am proud of my volunteer work accomplishments, and the feelings of achievement it has given me.

Retirement has proven beneficial because I remain active. It is wonderful to have the time to be able to help others—as I said before, not only does it give me a sense of personal satisfaction, but it keeps my mind off my own problems. I tell people, "Hey, I've had some good-bad luck! But, no matter what happens to you, always go on with your life."

I have known people who in turn have replied, "Hey, thanks a lot. I've never looked at the situation like that before."

Life is a trade-off of sorts. When things are going well, one takes much for granted. When things are going not so well, it is time to reflect on what is important to us. We all have some "good-bad" luck. The trick is to never give up, because, as soon as you do, the battle is over and you are defeated.

My retirement has also brought another dimension to my life, and one that many men never experience. And that, precisely, is a unique and special sense of awareness of my own family.

⊠⊠⊠⊠⊠⊠⊠⊠⊠⊠⊠⊠⊠⊠⊠⊠⊠⊠⊠⊠⊠

CHAPTER 12

There is not a day that goes by that I don't think about the benefits of having a solid marriage and wonderful family and the tremendous "plus" of having daughters—six of them to be exact. There is Karen, age 32; Debra, age 30; Kim, age 27; Donna, age 24; Diane, age 23; and Vickie, age 20.

Without a doubt, telling my family about my disease after it had been diagnosed was the hardest thing I have ever had to do. It took much soul searching on my part, as well as Shirley's, to find out the best way for us to tell the children what their father's medical problem was.

We explained the situation to them, being as honest and open as we possibly could, and made sure they understood that many of the severe symptoms an MS sufferer might experience may never happen to their father. While we did not "candy-coat" the problem, neither did we paint a portrait of doom and gloom. Only two of our children were old enough to fully understand at the time, but, on reflection, that was probably for the best.

Shirley and I have always been the type of parents who like to go to our children's events at school and attend functions they are involved in. I was determined never to let MS interfere with doing things with my kids. I wanted them to regard me as "normal" in every sense of the word and never be embarrassed by my MS. (I was also one of those outrageous parents who liked to participate in the kid's events, although I was not actually a member of any team. When they played soccer, I would occasionally run up and down the field, closely following the track of the ball. I would also yell—loudly! I think in retrospect that they were probably more embarrassed by their "fanatic" father's excitement than they ever were about MS.)

In relation to having daughters, one thought bothered me more than anything else, and I could not make light of it, nor could anyone convince me not to worry about it. I found myself wondering at times if I would be able to walk them down the aisle when they got married. However, I have been very fortunate in that I have been able to make that trip five times. Luckily, the wedding march is slow, which allowed me to do extremely well. (However, I do remember stepping on their gowns several times!)

It has struck me as amusing that on many occasions there was sort of a father-daughter role reversal going on behind the scenes. Can you picture the daughter being the one to steady the father instead of vice versa?

The father-daughter wedding dance was always short in my case. And, while I have often felt bad that I was not able to dance very well, I take much comfort in the fact that I was able to walk in the front door of the church.

My daughters were always there to do the things I could no longer do. When it reached the point where I could not climb stairs, they were right there to help me. Just to know I had someone to depend on if I needed it was reassuring—not that I could not do those things, mind you, but it was good to know I had a back-up.

When a family is close, it is said that the members automatically become "mind-readers," and this is exactly what has transpired over the years. My family helps me without even asking, making things so much easier for me. And, it is also true that adversity pulls a family closer together.

I have the tendency to experience radical mood swings, and this is probably the most perplexing thing for all of us to deal with. I wish I had a nickel for each time one of the girls would ask, "Dad, what's wrong?" There is usually nothing wrong—I am just going through a change of moods. I experience anger for no apparent reason, then strike out at my family in a display of emotion. I calm myself down at these times by realizing the frustration is toward myself rather than any of them.

Over the years, the family has tried to treat my health problems in a light and even humorous manner. Sometimes we have a good laugh at some of the antics I have pulled.

One evening we were seated at the table, awaiting the evening meal, talking about the day's activities as most families do. As we were talking, the salad dressing was passed to me and I proceeded to pour it on my salad.

However, it turned out that I missed my salad completely, dumping it all over my potatoes! As my coordination was bad and eyesight not up to par, I didn't realize what I was doing. The mistake was at my expense, but we all laughed about it together.

We were always so much better off laughing about these and other incidents, which might have been embarrassing to anyone else, rather than crying over them.

⌧⌧⌧⌧⌧⌧⌧⌧⌧⌧⌧⌧⌧⌧⌧⌧⌧⌧⌧

CHAPTER 13

I am sometimes plagued with feelings of self-pity. I ask, "Why me, Lord?"

Of course, at the same time, I have feelings of guilt mixed with gratitude in that I am not in a wheelchair and that I'm alive to see my family grow. There is a constant battle in my mind, between being grateful for what I do have and being angry for "getting stuck" with such a dreadful disease. I am always thankful that I am not fully incapacitated. And, again, the joy of having a supportive family certainly helps.

This leads me to a deeper subject—one most married couples have a hard time talking about—and that is the relationship between myself and my wife. Marriage is the ultimate commitment, and one that in this day and age is difficult to sustain even in the best of times.

When I was first told I had MS, I was ordered to give in to extra pressures of everyday life, such as running the family household, disciplining the children, and taking care of their needs. I also asked Shirley to start paying the bills, writing out checks at the end of the month, and so on. That was a powerful blow to the male ego, but it was something, under the circumstances, that needed to be done.

Of course, I had no doubt that she would do a fantastic job, but even this small task was hard to turn over. It had nothing to do with her ability. Rather, it had everything to do with my "maleness."

Shirley, on the other hand, was not the least bit resentful. In fact, she later told me she welcomed taking over the bill-paying duties, as I was always making such a mess out of things by making so many mistakes, and it was, in fact, easier for her to handle.

"I was happy to inherit the job," she had laughed. "The checkbook was always a mess and I viewed this as the chance to straighten things out."

When my eyesight was at a point where it was going downhill rapidly, Shirley took over the driving duties. Fortunately, she was and is an excellent driver, and I had no qualms about that. However, I suppose that I felt like most every other man would, in that it was hard for me to accept the facts of the situation. To let her do all the driving certainly was a hard shot at the old male ego!

I still drive, but only in uncongested areas with easy accessibility and only in those places that offer easy access to parking areas because of my bad eyesight. I do continue to drive whenever possible.

There is something I would like to touch on at this point. Although working women have become the norm in American society, I'm sure it had to be tough on Shirley to realize that while she was putting in 40 hours of work each week, I was on medical retirement and doing volunteer work, which paid nothing. I found a definite role reversal going on in the household. Shirley held the position of secretary at a bank during the day, and I stayed home and cleaned the house. She did not resent it, but I have to admit that I had my sensitive moments.

One day I remember cleaning the house from top to bottom and was awfully proud of my achievement. And, when Shirley arrived home that evening, I was quick to point this out.

"Look, dear," I said. "I dusted, washed all the dishes and vacuumed. Aren't you proud of the way the house looks?"

"Big deal!" was her reply.

My feelings were crushed. But one good thing to come out of it was that my retirement prompted me to purchase a dishwasher. It was a different story when I was the house-keeper, I can tell you that! (I will have to admit that I don't do windows or corners, nor do I move furniture, due to my health.)

⊠⊠⊠⊠⊠⊠⊠⊠⊠⊠⊠⊠⊠⊠⊠⊠⊠⊠⊠

CHAPTER 14

I have to say in all honesty that I am always appreciative of the fact that Shirley did not leave me when we found out I had MS. The marriage vows, to me, were in question, but at no time did she think about bailing out. This showed a tremendous amount of character on her part, and is one of the reasons I love her so much.

I felt guilty because I didn't want to saddle her down with a handicapped person the rest of her life. She, however, would hear none of it and refused to divorce me.

Upon retirement, I became much more attentive to family matters. Shirley was the disciplinarian when the children were small, and, because she was the one to take care of their needs, they naturally went to her with their problems.

I had a low level of patience when it came to the childish things they did (normal activities of every red-blooded child) and was quick to lose my temper on several occasions. However, as they got older, they began coming to me for advice. This was a gradual process and one that greatly improved with retirement.

Since I was retired, I had more "quality" time to spend with them—we were able to have lunch together often, as well as go on shopping trips. It became easier for them to confide in me, as I got to know them and their problems. It was also easier for them to confide in a father who wasn't upset with them all the time. Volunteer work helped in this area, as I would find myself thinking about my own children and relating those experiences to patients.

I also had a profound awareness of how fortunate I was to have my daughters. Every child reaches a rebellious stage in their teens, and my daughters were no exceptions. However, not once did they ever resent the fact that I had MS or show embarrassment. And, while doing volunteer work, I was also reminded time and again how seeing people in unfortunate situations makes one count their blessings.

My wife was understanding in other ways. During our marriage we slept in a double bed, until my health problems arose. Sometimes my legs jerk uncontrollably, which, at one time, caused my wife to lose a lot of sleep. She never complained, but after a few years of realizing this, I decided it would make it easier to switch to twin beds.

CHAPTER 15

So often it is easier to express oneself on paper rather than by spoken word. I have taken the liberty of offering letters that were written to me by members of my family, which have done so much in raising my spirits from time to time.

I would like to share them with you on the following pages.

Dearest David,

This particular letter, for me, is very difficult to write, only because for 20-odd years I have blocked my feelings as to how I honestly feel about you having MS. I felt that if I were actually honest with myself, that my anger, helplessness, and fury would surface and perhaps cause you to feel guilty, and in some way you might feel at fault for having this disease, and, possibly depriving your family in some way.

As it turns out, David, you are a very special man. There is determination and "get-up-and-go" that is unbelievable. You accept your "so-called disability" and in your own way give strength to your family.

This is not to say that we have not had problems. There are, of course, the ones that every family has with a half-dozen girls! And perhaps a few unique problems that only families with a husband, wife, or child with MS could understand.

Some of our difficulties are funny and humorous, and some could break your spirit if you did not really believe me and accept in your heart that indeed, "Tomorrow is a better day."

With all my love,
Shirley

To my father: David Atwood

Dear Dad,

You asked me to write down my thoughts and feelings when I found out that you had MS. I guess the best way to describe it is *angry*. I still am.

Not at you, at the disease.

I think that's because I don't understand it and that it happens to be you that has it!

If God is supposed to be so good, why are there diseases such as MS?

Why can't anything be done to help? Doctors can't fight it, so I believe the people who have it, *must*. I don't know how, that's why I'm angry.

I don't know if I have helped, but I hope so. I believe this book will help those with MS and those without.

I love both you and mother very much. And, Dad—I *can* read your writing!

All my love,
Kim

Dear Dad,

When I found out that my father had MS, I didn't know what to do or say. I also didn't know what it was or what it did to your body. My father would never show his pain.

My sisters and I would always see him do things like cut the grass in 100-degree weather and shovel the snow in 30-degree-below weather. We would say, "Don't do that, Dad!"

He would reply, "No!"

Dad, you loved doing things like that, so we let you. You would never sit down and relax, you were always on the go.

To this day, I wish there was a cure for MS. I know you would be first in line.

I love you and always will.

Love,
Donna

To Dad,

What is multiple sclerosis? You would be surprised at the number of people who don't know what those words mean. Oh, they may know that it's a disease, and it's something that someone else "catches."

Almost everything I know about MS I learned from you. You taught me what MS means: courage, faith, and never stopping. I think your main strength is trying to prove the doctors wrong—keeping one step ahead of the disease.

To me, MS is like a stack of blocks built underneath you. With every setback, the disease pulls out a few blocks. You topple some, regain your balance, then go on with life.

I'm sure there are days that you feel like staying in bed, pulling the covers over your head, and saying "the hell with it." But you don't—that's courage.

I guess you will never win any medals for your kind of courage. But, I know you don't care. You don't want medals—you have your family; and, in our eyes, you're a ten-star general.

I love you, Dad.
Karen

31

Dear Dad,

I am not very good at writing letters, but I will do my best. I don't really remember how old I was when I was told you had MS. I do know I never really understood why.

Why did my father have to get MS? I had a hard time accepting it; but, the more I looked at you and saw that nothing was going to stop you from doing what you wanted to, the easier it became for me. I have still always felt angry about it.

You have always been such a fighter. I am so glad you are not giving up on yourself. You are everything a person could ever want a father to be! I know you worried a lot about us girls being embarrassed about you, but I never was. I have always felt very proud, because you are a very strong-willed, loving, caring person. And I admire you greatly for this. I know it wasn't easy for you and Mom to raise six girls, but I think you have done a fantastic job. I hope you are both proud of me and what I have accomplished in my life so far. Dad, you still have one more trip down the aisle when I get married, even if it's five years from now.

I remember when we went fishing in the Ozarks. You couldn't walk on the docks to the boat—so you crawled. I thought that was great, because you got to the boat the best way you could. At least you didn't throw your hands in the air and say, "I can't do it."

If anything should ever happen to me, I pray that I have the courage and strength that you show every day of your life.

I love you and Mom very much, and I thank you both for everything. Dad, I have faith that there will be a cure for MS someday. I pray every night that someone will find a cure soon.

Dad, you are not fighting this battle alone—your family and friends are behind you all of the way!

Love,
Vickie Jo

Dear Dad,

I sit back thinking about how I feel about you having MS. I don't understand why it happened, and I guess I never will. I was pretty young when I first realized there was something wrong. You have always taken it so well. I don't know if I could have taken it as well or have been as strong.

You have always done whatever you could with us. I remember when Donna and I were on soccer and softball teams. You were always there, standing behind us. You would be up and down the sidelines right along with us. You were responsible for the tracks from one end of the field to the other. I know it hasn't been easy raising six girls. We had to have been, and still are, a handful.

When you and Mom found each other, it was a match made in heaven. Mom has understood and accepted the situation. I know the two of you have been through a lot. Dad, you have not let MS stand in your way. You have always given everything your best effort.

I'm afraid many people out there with MS sit back and let it get the best of them. You have always been one step ahead of it. Dad, do something for me. Stay the great father, husband, and strong person you have always been and don't let the MS ever get ahead of you.

We all pray one day very soon they will find a cure for this unfortunate disease that has entered the family. I will always stand behind you and do what I can to fight with you in the battle against MS. I love you and Mom!

Love,
Dee

Dear Dad,

I was fourteen years old when I first noticed any signs that there was anything wrong with you. I couldn't understand why you were wearing a patch over one of your eyes, why you seemed to be walking like you had been drinking all the time. I knew something was wrong, because you never did drink. It was then I found out that you had MS.

I did some reading about the way things happen with the balance and muscles with people with this most surprising illness. It seems to have most doctors shocked and puzzled. No matter how hard you tried to keep to yourself how you felt, we knew you were feeling poorly. We tried to get you to slow down—which was impossible!

You have helped me a lot and I owe you a very special thanks. The summer of 1971 was when I found out I was a diabetic. I always asked myself, "Why did this happen to me?" Then, one day, when I was in the hospital, I told myself to take a good look at you, with a disease nobody has a cure for. You were fighting it every day and doing very well. I then started looking on the bright side and started living and being happy.

There is a cure for diabetes, and we can lead happy, normal lives. Maybe someday there will be a cure for MS.

Dad, I pray someday things will look better for those with the illness. I'm here if you need me, because you were there when I needed someone. You made my life happier and brighter.

Love,
Debbie Trimble

CHAPTER 16

There is a familiar saying that "You can take the boy out of the country, but you can't take the country out of the boy."

I am, and always will be, a country boy. My roots, heart, and fondest memories belong to the country. There are many factors that go into molding a person's character. I will always be grateful for my rural upbringing and the strong, positive experiences that were a part of my childhood. The basic, solid values I was raised with have been invaluable to me over the years in withstanding physical difficulties I have had to face.

"Always help someone if you get a chance because you never know when you are going to need help yourself," was a philosophy I learned as a young boy and one that I have tried to follow all of my adult life. It is also a basic one. I know I have benefited from following that rule many times over the course of the years, being repaid in kind when the chips were down.

I was born in Naylor, Missouri—a small town situated

in the southeastern part of Missouri, way down in the foot-hills of the "Show-me" state—and lived there until the age of twelve. I jokingly tell people not to blink when passing through, or else they might miss it! It will probably come as a surprise to no one to know the population stands at 150.

My most cherished memories were formed not in the tiny town of my birth, however, but after my family moved to Oxley—another small farming town—located halfway between Naylor and Doniphan, Missouri.

My folks were farmers, and it was on the family farm that my brothers, Michael J. Atwood; sisters, Joyce Ann (Atwood) Jones and Mary Helen (Atwood) Jolly; and myself spent the next three years of our lives living the simple exist-ence of a farming family on a 368-acre spread.

Frank and Agness Atwood were hard workers. Dad was an intelligent and easygoing man; but, unfortunately he was not cut out to be a farmer. We later ended up selling the farm to make ends meet—a fact I still bemoan today.

Mother was the last of the great perfectionists. Her motto was, "If you've got a job to do, you damn well better do it right or don't do it at all."

This caring, intelligent woman lived her life by that say-ing. Mother had the dubious honor of handling the discipline of the children and "rules of etiquette" were strictly enforced throughout my childhood and adolescence.

I had a voracious appetite, and my favorite part of the day seemed to be when I got fed—just like one of the farm ani-mals. I had an insatiable appetite and actually looked forward to my next meal before I had finished the previous one, such was my enjoyment of mealtime. Mom always told me that my stomach would be the death of me someday. I can remember hoarding biscuits at dinner, hiding them under my plate as though I anticipated a severe famine across the country and making sure I would be ready for it.

I was not a troublemaker in school, nor was I ever the object of a scandal. However, I was just your basic, average kid when it came to hitting the books. I can honestly look back and say that at no point did I have a favorite subject in school. I did not discriminate—I didn't like any of them! I was definitely not crazy about being in school at *all*, and my happiest moments came each day when the schoolbell rang and I was dismissed. I was the type of kid who looked forward to summer vacation immediately after the Christmas vacation was over. It is a statement of fact to say that a scholar I was not!

Despite my lack of enthusiasm where school was concerned, I thoroughly enjoyed living on a farm. I would gladly choose daily chores over school any day. I became an old hand when it came to milking cows, picking cotton, and carrying wood. I may have had an ulterior motive to get the jobs done as quickly as possible, as I knew I would get to go horseback riding—my favorite sport and pastime—when I was finished.

It was on the farm that I learned to appreciate the little things in life—the good earth, the lovely sound of birds singing, the beauty of trees, and the peaceful sound of water rushing down a stream. I knew we were financially poor, but I was always happy, and the fact that I didn't have a lot of material things did not bother me in the least.

I can particularly remember summertime during those early years—sitting near the creekbed on a lazy afternoon. I might have done nothing more than sit and throw rocks on the water, my mind completely blank, but the peace and quiet was great. I loved to stand and look at a freshly plowed field— the image was comforting and soothing to a young boy like myself.

The crisis of my life came when the family was forced to sell the farm. I was at an impressionable age and being the wistful, romantic child that I was, took it hard. Stripping me of my horse was more than I could bear. My parents handled it quite well at the time and presented the transition as a fact of life. It was doing poor financially, and we had the choice to either move or starve. I believe the main reason I was able to deal with the upheaval was because I knew what was going on, and the reasons behind the move were explained to me clearly.

After leaving the farm, Dad went to work at McQuay Norris Ammunition plant as a factory worker. Mom took on double duty as a clerk at Kresge's and also worked as a book-keeper at Art Craft Venetian Blind Company in St. Louis.

I was seventeen years old when I went into the service. In those days, a person was expected to "put in time" in some branch of the armed forces, and it turned out to be my time to go. I was undecided about a career and did not like the idea of going to college, so the service seemed the natural place for me. My parents showed no reaction when I told them of my decision to go enlist. They signed all necessary legal papers, but it soon became clear that they didn't like the idea one bit— I was still their little boy as far as they were concerned.

I left my childhood fantasies behind upon entering the service, as well as a whole way of life. My innocence was lost.

I was to meet my future bride soon.

⌧⌧⌧⌧⌧⌧⌧⌧⌧⌧⌧⌧⌧⌧⌧⌧⌧⌧⌧⌧⌧

CHAPTER 17

My courtship of the former Shirley Steward began, appro-priately enough, when I was in the service. There was a neigh-borhood hangout called The Shamrock in Spokane, and by coincidence we both happened to be there one night. A mutual friend introduced us, and, as hokey as it sounds, I fell in love with her the first time I saw her.

She had big, brown eyes, so beautiful and expressive. Her features were attractive, and she had a lovely, slim figure. I asked her out to dinner immediately, but even before the big date, I knew she was special—and I knew I was hooked.

There were only two obstacles that stood in the way of our love affair: First, Shirley had no idea that I had fallen madly in love with her (and I later learned the feeling was not mutual) and therefore, did not acknowledge that she was ready to be whisked away by me. Second, I was engaged to another girl.

In my own defense, I would have to say that it was not unusual because I was *always* engaged to someone! In fact, my mother used to call me "Diamond Jim" because of my expensive tastes, which manifested themselves in my giving each girl I went out with for any length of time an engagement ring. Some guys give candy—I gave diamond engagement rings! It seems ludicrous when I remember having at least four rings sitting around the house—remnants of old relationships. (I should note that although I was nicknamed Diamond Jim. I did not have the wallet to go with my title. That fact alone made my expensive and ridiculous habit of bestowing diamond rings on ladies even more absurd.)

Shirley, on the other hand, found me to be a nice guy (more like "average") but certainly had no intentions of eloping after our first date. She had been married before and was extremely independent—she had to be with a family to raise. She was also hard-headed, a trait she calls "realistic." On her part, it was not a spontaneous moment, because she was not looking for a prince charming, like me, to sweep her off her feet.

In fact, I later learned that not only did she have the

audacity *not* to fall passionately in love with me, but she even felt I was somewhat immature.

"I remember thinking the situation you were in at the time as being so stupid," were her later reflections of the relationship. "Naturally, you were engaged, and your girl friend had sent you a red sucker in the shape of a heart for Valentine's Day. I remember taking it away from you and eating it myself! I also recall thinking you were immature, because it was such a ridiculous thing for people your age to do."

As I came to know Shirley, I was impressed by the way she took care of herself and three children by a previous marriage. She was a diligent, conscientious worker who supported her family by working as a bookkeeper during the day and a carhop at night. Her apartment was immaculate, and I found her personal stock to be very high. I admired her and respected her a great deal. Under those circumstances, I don't know if I could have done as well.

Through my dogged persistence, I finally won her over, and three months later we were engaged. And yes, I finally gave her an engagement ring—although I didn't present it to her until much later, at least not until after the second date!

Shirley confided in me that she thought of me as a caring, considerate person and loved the fact that I always brought her flowers whenever I saw her.

My parents were happy for us when it finally soaked in that I was actually—really and truly—going to marry her. My mother was a little apprehensive at first, concerned with the fact that it might be difficult because of the existing children. Shirley had a better grasp on this than I did and was not upset by her reaction. Later, my wife became as close to my mother as she was to her own.

My in-laws were terrific people. Mason and Gladys Stewart, Shirley's parents, offered much moral support as the years went by.

It used to make me wonder why Shirley's parents were always so willing to help me. After all, they didn't owe me anything and could just have easily tried to persuade their daughter to divorce her "handicapped" husband years ago.

They were true "Johnnys-on-the-spot" in times of crisis, offering help whenever needed. I cannot honestly say that I, as a parent, would have been as good.

CHAPTER 18

My early values played a large part in how I am able to cope with MS now. I actually saw my family get through rough times; and, after seeing things like that as a young boy, adolescent, and adult, I have been instilled with the strong desire to never give up and to appreciate the things in life that God has given me.

I know my mother had a lot to do with instilling my "push and drive." It seems like she was always sick with some sort of illness, but she never complained. Not even on the day she died.

I have early visions of her carrying a newborn calf up and down a steep hill to the creek so it could get a drink of water. I knew the whole time I watched that she was in physical pain.

I can also remember Grandfather Atwood, who died at the ripe old age of 92. The last few years of his life he crawled up and down the rows in his garden pulling out weeds. He had to crawl because his eyesight was so bad. But, it never once prevented him from living a full life.

Dad was 75 years old when he died from complications due to a bad heart. After his heart attack, he stopped working at his regular job but continued to thrive by doing the mowing, gardening, and other outdoor tasks. He, too, never stopped leading a full life.

To this day, I derive much strength from Shirley; watching her tackle the household duties and raise the children while keeping a full-time job never ceases to amaze me.

CHAPTER 19

It helps to know the facts about multiple sclerosis. I have referred to a pamphlet published by the National Multiple Sclerosis Society in many of my explanations, which I hope will shed light on the mysterious disease. I also hope people will gain an understanding of the problems we face.

Multiple sclerosis is a disease of the brain and spinal cord—it is one that affects the central nervous system as it interferes with the brain's ability to control normal bodily functions. Walking, speaking, seeing clearly, and even standing are things that a person with MS does not take for granted. These are the things that on any given day we might not be able to do.

To get an idea of how MS strikes, one should picture the central nervous system as one big switchboard that sends electrical messages along the nerves to different parts of the body. These messages control conscious as well as unconscious movements. MS blocks these messages by taking detours that lead to wrong areas and by not getting through correctly. (Most healthy nerve fibers are insulated by *myelin*, a fatty substance that aids the flow of messages. In MS, the myelin breaks down and is replaced by *slera*, or scar tissues. This is what distorts or even blocks the flow of messages.

But the problems associated with MS are not necessarily the one I have listed above, which to an ordinary person might seem the most obvious.

The worst thing about MS is that it is a disease that is totally unpredictable, making it impossible to plan for the future.

On some days, the symptoms might be so mild that, while they are noticeable and rather annoying, it is still possible to proceed with a normal daily routine. Then there are the "in-between" days. Those are the times when the symptoms are somewhat pronounced, and the old body just is not functioning up to par. However, with proper care and a little juggling of priorities, I can still go about getting things done.

And then there are the "black" days. When I hit one of those days, it just doesn't pay to get out of bed! On those days, I may experience one or all of the symptoms in such a severe form that it becomes impossible to plan any kind of a daily routine.

You never really know when the symptoms of MS will strike. As I've pointed out, I may get struck with one, two, or all of the symptoms on any given day: eye trouble, speech problems, partial or complete paralysis, extreme weakness, shaking of hands, loss of coordination, loss of bladder (or bowel) control, numbness, staggering, loss of equilibrium, and dragging of feet.

Typically, the symptoms start out mild and then may disappear. (This is how I was initially affected—believe me, the disease is a trick player!)

Early symptoms, because they are so slight, may go unnoticed, only to reappear and become more numerous and severe in later years. There are lucky MS patients, who have had the disease go into remission early and remain so. And, there are also the unlucky ones, who have been hit severely in the beginning, with the disease remaining that way, even becoming bedridden for long periods of time. You just never really know. . . .

It is believed that, based on research, the disease most often occurs to people living in temperate zones between forty and sixty degrees north and south latitudes. The closer an area to the equator, the fewer the cases of MS. Children in areas not exposed to some factors that might help build an immunity to MS may also become afflicted.

CHAPTER 20

There are numerous theories as to what causes MS and who the people are that most likely will get it. But theories remain just that—only theories, and not scientific fact. I'm sure, like myself, people with MS can point to a particular theory and claim it as their own.

I have had many years to think about it and to speculate as to how I happened to contract the disease. Therefore, I have come up with my own special hypothesis.

I believe I contracted a virus while in the service (1957) stationed at a radar site in Saglak Bay, Labrador, in a northern province of Canada. The site, situated on top of a 1400-foot-high mountain, was located on the bank of the North Atlantic, a few hundred miles off Thule, Greenland.

In the winter, the temperature reached ten degrees below zero and less. High, raging winds were normal. It was also unusual for a Midwestern boy like myself to sit through twenty-four hours of darkness on winter days, and twenty-four hours of daylight during the summer months.

During the winter, on that particular site, our waterline broke one day. There were about eighty people on that site, and it was during that time that I picked up the virus that later caused MS. I also wonder how many, if any, other people contracted the disease.

The theories scientists have come up with include virus attacks, such as the one I described, as a possible link with MS. They also point to a theory of immune reactions, as well as a theory that includes a combination of both. I personally believe it was a slow-acting, delayed reaction to a common virus I picked up while there.

I must point out that this theory is strictly personal. It is true that when something bad happens to you, it is natural to search for answers—and that includes grasping at straws if necessary. My headaches, as well as my left eye turning outward, were the first signs of MS. They occurred the following year, and this is the conclusion I have drawn.

It may or may not be correct. As I said, we all have the tendency to devise our own ways of thinking when we have a disease that cannot be explained—in this case, MS.

CHAPTER 21

A person with MS is advised to keep himself or herself as healthy as possible, and that includes what I consider the most important factor—namely, keeping a positive mental attitude.

Any doctor, it would stand to reason, would offer this advice to any patient; but, with MS sufferers, it is extremely important.

A nutritious diet, adequate rest, and a reasonable amount of exercise to ease the tightening of muscles has been recommended to me. As I stated earlier, we have no definite clue as to what causes the disease and how it will progress. It stands to reason that there is no cure available, given all the "unknowns" involved.

Patients may be given vitamins to help make sure they are receiving the proper nutrients. They may also be given muscle relaxers to relieve possible muscle spasms; and, hormones may be prescribed to help reduce the severity of attacks. But, there is no pill available to make the disease go away; medication and a reasonable health plan, however, will help relieve specific symptoms.

There are a number of outside factors that affect me. I believe the climate plays a large part in how I function. The fall and spring seasons are, without a doubt, the best times for me, both mentally and physically. My balance is steadier, and during these periods I always have an optimistic attitude and view on life. I also feel more confident in my abilities. I can sum it up by saying that I have "peace of mind."

I function best in the morning and often wish "mornings" would last all day! Around noon, I tend to slow down. Again, the way I react to each day depends on the severity of the symptoms on that particular day.

My emotional health is something I have learned to put a high premium on. When my emotions run high and I am angry or upset, my sense of balance suffers and my speech takes a turn for the worst. The end result is increased stuttering and slurring of words. Symptoms of MS that I have not experienced in past months tend to hit me when I become emotional.

I remember a conversation with a woman I met one morning at the restaurant I frequent. I noticed she relied on the use of a walker with every step she took, and for some strange reason, I was curious if she might have MS.

I learned that she did indeed suffer from it. She told me that her mother had died recently, and because of her poor mental and emotional health, she found it harder to function physically. Hence the walker.

I related to what she was saying. In the course of meeting MS patients, we find we aren't alone in these emotional situations. Morale encouragement from others comes in handy at times like these.

I know there are times when I resemble a zombie, showing no reaction. However, I still "feel" like everyone else— I just try harder to keep my emotions in check.

Many people don't know how to deal with a person, be it friend or relative, that has MS. This is understandable, but the fears are groundless and often make us even more self-conscious.

The woman with the walker said that when she told people she had MS, they always looked at her strangely. This response is common; but, believe me, we are normal people— we just have physical problems.

MS is not contagious, nor is it a form of mental illness. An MS sufferer may exhibit erratic behavior at times—such as walking as though intoxicated or abruptly losing balance— but it is important to remember that we cannot control this. It is a disease of the central nervous system, and thus we have no control over our movements.

It is a constant struggle for me to keep a positive mental attitude. It is also a struggle to maintain a low frustration level and live with the idea that I won't give in to self-pity. It keeps me going knowing that I owe it to myself and my family not to feel sorry for myself.

I feel pressure in so many ways. I feel pressure not to accidentally lose my balance and fall, knocking things over in gift shops; I feel pressure not to fall down when stepping onto a curb, and I feel pressure to enunciate clearly over the telephone. I know about these pressures ahead of time and always make a concerted effort to overcome them in advance.

Even the small tasks pose difficult challenges for MSers.

There are a number of ways my morale can be boosted. Some of the things that help me deal with MS include talking to other people who have the disease and relating with them incidents that occur throughout the day. I also enjoy frequenting places where there are people I know who are familiar with my problems. It is comforting to know that assistance and help will be offered without explanation. My favorite hangout is a neighborhood restaurant located in a supermarket. I like to know that I can sit down and enjoy a meal without feeling like I'm on pins and needles.

At Schnuck's Grandview Restaurant (located in Florissant, Missouri), I have spilled a few glasses of water, dropped a number of biscuits, and lost my balance en route to the parking lot. However, the waitresses and cooks understand my problems, as do the "regulars" who frequent the place. Just knowing there is a spot where I can relax and feel comfortable gives my spirit a great lift every day. It helps to keep a good mental attitude when I surround myself with supportive people.

I also like to set new goals for myself. I was overcome with an enormous sense of accomplishment when I gave a speech in front of fifty people at an MS support group meeting in May 1985. All systems were go—I spoke clearly, my nerves were kept under control, and I was able to stand straight.

It took me four years to reach the point where I even thought about attempting this.

"Gratifying" is the only word I can use to describe this milestone in my life.

🞨🞨🞨🞨🞨🞨🞨🞨🞨🞨🞨🞨🞨🞨🞨🞨🞨🞨🞨

CHAPTER 22

MS patients lead normal lives. We have the same day-to-day problems: raising our families, getting the bills paid, and determining where to spend our summer vacations.

We also have to deal with unexpected medical problems like anyone else. However, when we develop additional medical problems, it is like one foot of snow falling over two inches of ice! The situation is compounded.

I first began experiencing heart problems in 1973. My heartbeat had been irregular, and it was a condition that gradually became aggravating. After consulting a heart specialist at Barnes Hospital, I was told my heart was *fibulating*. It was a minor condition that had the potential to become serious. Fortunately, it straightened itself out, and I was spared further complications.

The initial tests showed that my heart was beating normally. I was thankful for this. By this time I was so accustomed to staying in hospitals that I didn't think there was anything left to scare me. I was wrong! The tests proved unnerving. I was put in a state of helplessness; stretched flat on my back on a cold, hard slab, and hooked up to a machine. I could exert no control over my environment and therefore felt plain scared. The only comfort was the steady beat of the heart monitor.

Life was smooth sailing until the summer of 1974. I was

49

mowing the lawn one day when a peculiar feeling overcame me. I became more tired than usual, which, ordinarily, I would have chalked up to MS. I was used to dealing with poor health on a fairly regular basis and, naturally, tried to brainwash myself into thinking this was just a usual problem. However, this time the feeling was very pronounced. I continued to cut grass, feeling as though I was carrying a ton of bricks on my shoulders. Each movement was forced. I began to experience discomfort down the middle of my back and shortness of breath. I stopped at that point only because I had finished cutting the entire front yard. I sometimes speculate about the end result had I continued to push myself.

The next day the family doctor took an EKG and sent me directly to the hospital. It was determined, after tests, that I had suffered a heart attack and was to remain in the hospital for two weeks.

My mother, father, and uncle had been plagued with heart problems, so there was a family history. Mine was brought on by *arteriosclerosis*, the thickening and hardening of the inner walls of the heart, impairing the circulation of the blood. Thank God it was minor. I was told to take life easy for a while, to gradually build up my strength, and to come in for weekly checkups.

My sense of balance worsened after the heart attack and stayed that way for months. However, I was told there was no connection between the attack and MS.

Small projects kept me busy during the recuperation period. I did research on the history of some very old gold leases that belonged to my mother, and I also spent time painting. After the normal recuperation period, Shirley and I took a much-needed vacation.

In 1977, it was determined that I was suffering from *vasculitis*, a condition where one component of the blood reacts with another component, causing change. It appeared as a rash, causing me to break out in red bumps all over my body. In my case, the bumps ranged from small to large; sometimes they would be isolated, while other times there would be many of them.

That particular year was not one of my better ones. I lost ten pounds that summer, which was a significant weight loss for someone of my build. This alarmed me, prompting a visit to the family doctor.

Prednisone, an oral steroid, had been prescribed for the vasculitis but, unfortunately, masked symptoms of another malady. I was told that I had dormant tuberculosis. I was taken off the medication long enough to obtain a positive diagnosis.

Finding out what the problem was, at the time, a tedious process that took a conscientious doctor leading the way.

Luckily, I went through only one treatment for tuberculosis, and tests were negative. I was given a clean slate of health and resumed the Prednisone shortly thereafter. After the heart attack I had been put on a strict diet but was now told to eat anything I wanted, to put some weight back on—thank God for small favors!

I have also had a condition known as *optic neuritis* in my left eye for thirty years. It is a condition where the optic nerve of the eye becomes inflamed, causing blurred vision. While it is not connected with MS, it has added to my medical problems over the years.

Before I leave the problem of my health behind, I would like to say that I wear a medic alert tag at all times. It is important for outsiders to know that I have MS so they know what to do in case of an emergency. I also appreciate people knowing I am not a drunk, should they happen to see me staggering somewhere!

CHAPTER 23

Human sexuality is a subject that has bombarded the public for the past few years. I believe every married couple has had its share of sexual problems brought on by a variety of factors—sometimes physical, sometimes not.

There have been problems of a sexual nature in our marriage, but there is no way that blame can be placed strictly on the physical aspect of MS.

It is true that, in males, suffering from MS may cause occasional impotency problems. However, the extent of this condition varies greatly from one individual to another. I would also like to add that this is a normal occurrence and should be dealt with as such.

Unfortunately, it was difficult to put that into its proper perspective, and my attitude gradually became one of "if I wasn't able to perform right, it must be *her* fault."

This is the defense mechanism we sometimes rely on if things aren't going right; we have to find someone else to put blame on—we sure aren't going to blame ourselves, are we? (As with trying to come up with a personal theory for the cause of MS, here too, we like to grasp at straws.)

But "blame" isn't the correct terminology. MS is a disease for which there can be no blame, and, consequently, symptoms are likewise.

I had so many fears in the back of my mind. I feared Shirley would judge *me* by the symptoms of MS—symptoms over which I had no control; I feared the symptoms would completely take over, causing us both frustration and embarrassment; and, I feared she would leave me.

When I realized how stupid my fears really were, and how selfish and self-centered I had become, I was able to deal with the real problem. I have long since found there is much more to "making love" than the physical act alone.

⌧⌧⌧⌧⌧⌧⌧⌧⌧⌧⌧⌧⌧⌧⌧⌧⌧⌧⌧

CHAPTER 24

It has been eighteen years since I was diagnosed as having multiple sclerosis. I have done my best to try and share with you my experiences in dealing with the disease, as well as to provide insight into how my family and friends have dealt with it over the years.

Tomorrow Is a Better Day has proven to be a perfect title for the book. Speaking from the voice of experience, I can assure you that there is always a better tomorrow! It does not matter if "better" means just getting up and being able to stand on your own two feet—to me, that is an accomplishment. I have learned to take each day at a time and make the best of what God has given me.

I sincerely hope the experiences presented in this book will shed light on MS and make it easier for those afflicted to have hope and confidence in themselves and faith in God. I am convinced that someday a cure will be discovered for the disease; but, until that day comes, I do not intend to give up!

Hopefully, all men and women can learn from my mistakes, whether they have MS or not.

Never blame your partner for your problems; never quit trying to give and receive love; and, never withhold affection from your partner for any reason!

⌧⌧⌧⌧⌧⌧⌧⌧⌧⌧⌧⌧⌧⌧⌧⌧⌧⌧⌧

CHAPTER 25

Tragedy is also something we MSers cannot escape, nor can we protect our loved ones from it.

The saddest period in our lives came when we lost our only son, David Lee Atwood, Jr. Shirley had given birth to this tiny, helpless baby on July 15, 1963; his death followed on August 8, 1963—only three short weeks later.

The pregnancy was, by all indications, a normal one. Since he was Shirley's sixth child, neither of us thought there would be complications.

A reversed heart was determined as the cause of death. Twenty-two years ago, a limited type of heart surgery was available; it could not compare with the strides being made today. David, Jr., didn't make it home—he died in the hospital.

We had the highest hopes for his recovery; but, in the back of our minds, we had doubts the infant would make it. We experienced deep depression; but Shirley was the one who coped with it much better than I.

She and her mom were the ones to go to the funeral home and pick out the casket. I had the feeling that somehow I was responsible. Doctors told me there was absolutely no connection between his condition and MS. I believed them but still felt guilty.

When an adult family member or loved one is dying, both parties generally prefer the patient stay in his or her own home, surrounded by familiar people and surroundings.

The opposite feeling was true for us, and it reminds me of my "good-bad" luck. It's bad he had to die, but good we didn't have to experience the agony of seeing him in his room and knowing we would never have the privilege of watching him grow up. We also knew that he was receiving the best care possible.

No matter what happens to you in this lifetime, you will always be able to look around you and find those in worse positions. That is why I say: Appreciate life, take each day as it comes, and thank the good Lord that you are alive to see it.

ⅩⅩⅩⅩⅩⅩⅩⅩⅩⅩⅩⅩⅩⅩⅩⅩⅩⅩⅩ

CHAPTER 26

FACT SHEET

Name: David Lee Atwood   D.O.B. 12/15/38

Address: 622 Hunters Ridge

City State ZIP: Ferguson, Missouri 63135

High school: Soldan Blewett High (Class of 1956)

Other: University of Missouri, St. Louis (1961 and 1962)

Military Service: U.S. Air Force

Years: 1956–60 (Honorable discharge)

Religion: Catholic

Occupation: Chemical research technician

Employed: Monsanto Company (1960–81)

Rating: Double-A Plus (1974)

Hobbies: Swimming, fishing, hunting, and horseback riding,
at one time. Volunteer work at hospitals and Red
Cross.

Date of diagnosis: Summer of 1958 (First noted, not positive)

Hospital: Letterman Army Hospital, San Francisco, California

Reoccurred: Summer of 1967 (Age 29)

Medical Retirement: March 31, 1981

Doctors: Dr. Lawrence Lawton, M.D. (first family doctor)

Dr. Henry Lattinville, M.D. (May 3, 1968)

Dr. Richard Ferry, M.D. (reconfirmed MS diagnosis)

Medical Schedule: Dr. Lawrence sent me to see Dr. Lattinville, then to Dr. Ferry.

Treatment: Short courses of Cortisone therapy, vitamin B-12
shots by Dr. Lawton, later by Dr. Tanphichitr;
5–15 mg of Prednisone daily, and vitamins.

Marriage: April 27, 1959

Wife

Name: Shirley Ann Atwood   D.O.B. 8/20/35

Maiden name: Stewart

High school: Tilgman High School

Hometown: Paducah, Kentucky

Occupation: Executive secretary and word processer

Company: Landmark Bank

Religion: Baptist

Hobbies: Playing cards, attending to family needs, and TLC

Children

(First three by Shirley's previous marriage)

1. Karen Lynn Trimble Atwood   D.O.B. 9/24/52

2. Debra Ann Trimble Atwood   D.O.B. 10/27/54

3. Kimberly Rae Trimble Atwood   D.O.B. 2/8/56

4. Donna Marie Atwood   D.O.B. 2/19/60

5. Diane Lynn Atwood   D.O.B. 3/20/61

6. David Lee Atwood, Jr.   D.O.B. 7/15/63
                                                  (Died 8/5/63)

7. Vickie Jo Atwood   D.O.B. 12/24/64

David Atwood's Parents

Father: Frank J. Atwood (deceased) D.O.B. 12/31/09

Mother: Agness Marian Atwood (deceased) D.O.B. 9/22/11

Residence: Florissant, Missouri

Shirley Atwood's Parents

Father: Mason Evans Stewart D.O.B. 10/17/14

Mother: Gladys Hope Shephard Stewart D.O.B. 11/14/16

Residence: O'Fallon, Missouri

POSTSCRIPT

I mentioned that tragedy was something that MSers cannot escape and must now add yet another unfortunate event to which we were not immune.

I regret to add that my wife and I were divorced on August 19, 1985, after twenty-six years of marriage.

Divorce is not a pleasant thing, no matter how one looks at it, and it will go down as one of the saddest experiences of my life. Yet divorce is a part of life and one that many of us must cope with. We have six beautiful daughters, whom we are proud of, and good memories that we have shared; and for that I am grateful.

No one can predict divorce in a crystal ball any more than I could have predicted that I would contract MS at a certain age. However, the important thing is how we cope with life's uncertainties, and I am confident that all of us will weather the storm—just as we have done in the past.